# Healing Our Community

## For Use at the United Nations, and in the U.S.A.

## Real Community Healing

## Heal Our Communities - Heal Our Nation - Heal Our World

**Published by:**

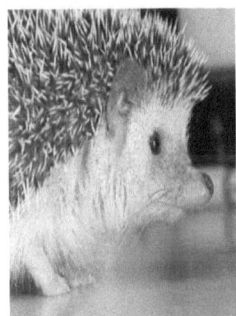

**Healing Hedgehog Press**
Cupertino, California   95014

healingangelguides@yahoo.com
**Email us today.**

**Web Site with TV shows, trainings, and testimonials.**
www.healingangelguides.com
**(408) 253-6577**  Office Phone

**ISBN-13: 978-1495281457**

**ISBN-10: 1495281450**
**BISAC: Health & Fitness / Healing**

**First Edition**

# Good News!

This is a group healing process that allows you to heal an entire group, regardless of the size of the group. Anyone can learn to do this process with small or large groups. It is deliberately written to make it easy to understand. There is no need to wait any longer to work toward world peace. You read from a list of actions or statements, and have the group do those actions. Past group trauma is handled/balanced, people leave feeling better, and there can be a shift in personal and community energy.

This process is real. This process works. Traumatic societal events that have happened globally get stuck in the group consciousness. Wars, terrorist attacks, bombings, gang violence, mass slayings, genocide, enslavement, and dictatorial control of peoples lives, etc. creates group trauma. This is the first process of this kind that can neutralize this group trauma regardless of the size of the group.

Call a group of your friends, try it and see for yourself.

Real community healing is within your grasp.

This is a first on planet Earth.

We invite you to think of the possibilities.

# Other Books by Paul Barbaro

**Heart to Heart Healing** – Getting Rid of Early Childhood Trauma. When you care enough to make a difference in a loved one's health. This imbalance resolves over time, just like a battery running out of energy through attached jumper cables.

**Healing Our Company** – Real Healing for a Troubled Workplace – Team Building that Heals

**Angelology** – The Quest for a better connection with Universal Mind.

**Two Shamans and a Healer** – The Quest for a Healing Discovery and, An Outline for a PBS Special

**The Lightbearers Handbook** – Let Your Light Shine Brighter

# You Can Be the Healing that
# You Want to See in the World!

This book is written for those frustrated individuals who want to do something to speed up the healing of our communities, states, nations and ultimately the world.

When our group pain is balanced, neutralized, and healed, we make different decisions as a society. This is good.

This is how we will evolve from fear and greed to charity/generosity and love/care/concern.

A lasting world peace is now within our grasp. What we need is thousands of community healing groups meeting weekly to do this process and shift the energy of the earth. Yes. It will take a lot of us.

Rome was not built in a day and it requires work to turn this ship around. It took eons of shared community pain to put us into this position. It will take some work and time to completely heal. You and we are worth the work it takes to correct our course.

This process is written out verbatim to make it easy to do. With this book in hand, get a group of people together, and get the groups agreement to do the process. Then read a line from this book, have them say it to their partner, read another line and have the group do/say it until all the lines are done. As we do the process together, we heal as a group. This process was deliberately made easy to do. All the complexity of healing energy has been removed.

This process works because the healing energy goes around and around the circle, and it is as if all the people in the group are working on each other. There is a tremendous blessing for taking responsibility for helping heal ones' "tribe" community, state, nation and world. The larger the group, the greater the energy.

Editors Note: One can see FREE training videos of this technique at www.healingangelguides.com/  Please click on "Training" and watch these videos with a friend or partner, read this book together and then take turns doing this process on each other, One can get a result while doing the exercises. The gains can be tremendous.

## Youtube Videos that You can watch Online;

Youtube address for Video #1;
**http://www.youtube.com/watch?v=M_CdVe-_qsY**

Youtube address for Video #2;
**http://www.youtube.com/watch?v=FE-aNtbuqlk**

Youtube address for Video #3;
**http://www.youtube.com/watch?v=XunCrduVOto**

# Disclaimer

**Required Disclaimer:** The information provided in this book is for educational and entertainment purposes only and is not intended to diagnose, prevent, cure, nor treat any disease or condition. It is not intended as a substitute for competent medical care or advice. If one has pain then one is advised to see a medical professional immediately. If one is under a doctor's care, one must get their doctors permission to receive these energy healing processes. The information provided herein should not be construed as a health-care diagnosis, treatment regimen or any other prescribed health-care advice or instruction. The information is provided with the understanding that the publisher and author is not engaged in the practice of medicine or any other health-care profession and does not enter into a health-care practitioner/patient relationship with its readers. The publisher and author do/does not advise or recommend to its readers treatment or action with regard to matters relating to their health or well-being other than to suggest that readers consult appropriate health-care professionals in such matters. No action should be taken based solely on the content of this publication. The information and opinions provided herein are believed to be accurate and sound at the time of publication, based on the best judgment available to the author. However, readers who rely on information in this publication to replace the advice of health-care professionals, or who fail to consult with health-care professionals, assume all risks of such conduct. The publisher and author is/are not responsible for errors or omissions.

These statements have not been evaluated by the Food and Drug Administration. This product or process is not intended to diagnose, treat, cure, or prevent any disease.

If one has pain then one is advised to see a medical professional immediately. If one is under a doctor's care, one must get their doctor's permission to receive these energy healing processes.

Pain is symptomatic. Always seek medical advice from your physician or other qualified healthcare provider for any questions one may have regarding any medical condition including pain. And under no circumstances discontinue taking any prescribed medications without your doctor's permission. There are life threatening major diseases and medical conditions that have no symptoms at all. Regularly scheduled medical checkups are extremely valuable.

**More Disclaimer:** I, Paul Barbaro, created this spiritual work is a complement to conventional medicine and alternative healing methods. I'm a minister and this spiritual energy work is not a substitute for conventional medical treatment of any kind, physical or psychological. For such issues you should seek the proper licensed physician or qualified health care professional. This energy work may help the bio-field to come into energetic balance. Qigong theory believes when one's energy field is in balance, the body's latent healing ability can heal itself. I make no promises nor guarantees about the results of this work. I am very grateful for this opportunity to work with everyone interested in healing. I, Paul Barbaro, make absolutely no promises, because every body is different and everybody responds differently to healing energy. "Viva la difference."

**Notice:** This healing method revives the ancient and traditional "hands-on healing method" as spoken of in the Jewish sacred writings and in the Christian Bible, and uses the Buddhist, Hindu, Vedic, and Judeo-Christian teachings and upon the religious teachings of; "Do unto others as you would have them do unto you." It is also based on Chinese Ti-Chi, the movement of energy, and on Qui Gong, and other Asian and First American Nation (American Indian) energy religious and spiritual practices. Heart to Heart Healing University, Cupertino, California, is an ecclesiastic* educational association organized under the authority of the First Amendment of the Original United States Constitution, of the year of Our Lord 1789. This University is religious, it is a church university, and these healing processes are religious because they resolve spiritual stuck energy as well as the cellular memory of early physical trauma. All First Amendment rights are asserted, reserved, and protected herewith by this Notice, assertion, proclamation, and publication. The University is non-denominational, non-medical, and non-political. It is open to all races, creeds and religions, as well as to all sexual orientations. This healing University is not exclusive nor discriminatory. This is because we all can use some healing.

This healing method and these processes are not based on the belief systems of either the giver nor the receiver. It operates at the cellular level. It can repair damaged nerve connections at the cellular level. It can repair/forgive past ancestor's health issues. Belief systems, thought processes, spiritual orientation or lack thereof, and skill level of the giver are not a part of these processes. These processes are rote, and the results are rote. One simply does the process as taught. The results flow from there. This author has not found a person that these processes can not benefit. Whether the giver or receiver "feels" anything or not is irrelevant. This is a "balance energy" process, not a 'feel' process. Balance can not do harm. Some people feel nothing, for others the earth shifts under their feet and their whole life goes smoothly, easier, "better" or differently. This process is subtle. It looks simple and runs deep. Please see the section on detox reactions for more information.

**Note:** These processes are not instant. There are no magic bullets. There are no magic pills.

As Rome was not built in a day, and as your immune system is/was not instantly compromised, so these processes take time and work to achieve long lasting results. You and your partner are worth the work. You both are worth the time spent, and you are both worth working toward the results.

No claims of results can ever be made from these processes because every body and every trauma is different, and heals differently. Some chronic pain does not respond to balanced energy, one is always free to explore other avenues of healing.

Just for clarity, there is no suggestion that there is anything wrong with the reader, their families nor friends, nor any of our societies. We are all made perfectly. There is nothing wrong with you or anyone or anything else. To judge this would be an injustice to the judged. This authors goal is to help "Turn up the/your 'Light' a little brighter." Not that it's dim. Thank you for your understanding.

# Table of Contents

# Who Are We? And,

# Where did We Come From?

We at the Heart to Heart Center have been resolving early childhood pain/trauma since 2008 in San Jose, California. This author thought he was "pretty good" as a healer until two First Nation (Native American Indian) Shamans straightened him out.

We teach that when one thoroughly understands where pain comes from, it is not difficult to resolve it. Once early childhood pain is balanced, the later negative health issues are extinguished. In other words; "Once your early childhood pain is balanced, systems in your body work better. And your body knows how to heal itself."

Balance and flow is good for your body. You can balance an unbalanced system. You can balance early child trauma and start your healing, even years after the events. Happy balancing and healing to you! The story of Paul Barbaro's healing enlightenment is found in two of his books; "Heart to Heart Healing," and "Two Shamans and a Healer." Both books are available from Amazon.

## Healing Entire Groups

Our later research provided us with discoveries that allow us to heal entire groups of people thus speeding up healing on Earth. This is good for world peace which is now within our reach. All we need is dedicated groups of people around the world doing this process weekly and negative the energy will shift to positive.

# Acknowledgements

First of all I wish to acknowledge my wonderful life mate, Adriana Steinwedel, my entire Barbaro, Gironda, and Ryland/Nomura tribes, as well as the Hollar, Montes, Caballero, Castillo, Garcia, Rodreguez, Mendoza, Flores, Rivera, Alvarez, Gomez, Diaz, Reyes, Morales, Robles, Moreno, Cortez, Romero, Agulara, Ramerez, Torres, Hernandez, and all other supporting tribes, clans, and families. And all the health pioneers that so bravely stepped out to tell the truth; Dr. M. Oz, Dr. Deepak Chopra, Dr. C. Everett Koop, Dr. Andrew Weil , Dr. Sears, Gregg Braden, Carolyn Myss, Carol Sutherland, David Wilcock, Nick Delgado, Dr. Wayne Dyer, Dr. Bruce Lipton, Michael Bernard Beckwith, Jacqueline, Marianne Williamson, Louise Hay, Dr. Carl Ferreri, DC, David Wolf, John Gray, Sounds True, Hay House, and all the hundreds of other alternative health leaders.

I have such gratitude, admiration and hope for the possibility of success for world peace. With this healing method, world peace is possible because group pain can be eliminated.

# Healing Our Community
# with The Healing Circle

## Forward

Please realize that this Group healing has never existed on Earth before now in this easy to learn, and easy to do form. Today, this is a chance to make a real positive impact on our communities, our leaders and our lives.

If you like how things are going here on Earth, there is no need do this process. Lucky you!

You have this unique opportunity to become the healing you want to see in the world.

And, "Yes!" You can do this even if you have a day job and two children, and you are a very busy person! And you can do this process even if you have no or little healer training nor know much about energy and energy healing.

We as a species are overdue for this group healing process. I support a healing shift in community energy.

When you arrive at the knowledge that this process works, and you are willing to rise to be the healing you want to see in the world, this process is a gem of an aid in making a change in your community and in the world. An added benefit is that as you help others heal, you also experience healing yourself. It is truly a toss up as to who gets the most out of this healing work.

# Healing A Group, Producing a Shift

This book is an answer to healing large numbers of people all at the same time. This is cutting edge healing and this is the future of healing. It is highly desirable to speed up the healing of our cultures, societies, church congregations, political bodies, civic organizations, clubs, family and groups of friends and acquaintances, etc..

Understanding this healing process is power. When the energy of the people shifts, the energy of the world will shift. We are overdue for that shift.

Note: This is not an instant process. It requires work. It requires sharing this process with hundreds of groups all over the world. That's why this author needs lots of willing healers to step up to the challenge to make a real difference in the world. It's all energy and it can shift and change with this process.

For those of you that are waiting for our leaders to do this for us. Give it up! They are so dysfunctional that they simply will never evolve to that responsibility. So it is up to you and me. It's a tough job but someone has got to do it. Let's roll up our sleeves and get it done.

# Healing Circle Outline

**Rule #1;** Don't believe anything I say. Experience it, feel the results, then believe it, and help others learn to do it!

Rule #2; Change nothing, ever. Read the instructions, starting at the top of page number 12 to the group exactly as it is written for the best results. This process works very well. Reading from a book makes it easy and comfortable to do. You don't need to be a public speaker. This is good news. What is needed is for the group to be willing to work for their betterment, and to be willing to do the process by following your instructions. Your part is to read a line from this book and have them do the action as best they can. You can coach them as to how to do it. After you do this process with two to three groups you will feel comfortable and be able to do it anywhere and with any group. We are always open to suggestions. Please email us any insights or thoughts that may make this a more effective process.

Let's Imagine Together! Let's Invite Your Angels, Ancestors, Masters, Guides, Saints, Friends & Family, & All the Great Healers of all time to be in this room now, and to help with your healing. And they are invited to heal together with us.

We will invite the Archangels Michael, Gabriel, Uriel, and Raphael – also known as "The Healer," and all the other angels.

We address the stuck energy of your ancestors because it may have killed them. That energy which took them out is still in your DNA! You are so spiritually and DNA connected to your ancestors, relatives, family that even if you don't know them, nor can you care about them, they are key to your healing, like them or not. Just do the process. It works.

Past and future generations are getting healed here today, right now! How will that impact your life when that stuck energy is released, and people are free?

These processes are not just a "Nice Theory"! They work! These processes work on every person every time. This author does not write anything that does not work 100% of the time on 100% of the people! Every person is different and every body perceives healing differently. That's the difference! Even if you or your partner feel nothing, the process still cuts to the bone of the trauma!

## Your Ancestor's Greatest Fear

Your ancestor's greatest fear is that they will be forgotten. They did not live their lives and work hard to be forgotten. This strikes terror in their hearts. An entire genetic line of theirs dying out is a tragedy of great proportion because that line can never be re-created.

# This is an Audience Participation Event

**A Guarantee:** If you participate fully and give 100% of your effort in this next hour you will have a shift in your body's energy for the better.

That does not mean that you are done with the balancing process. You may require more work because other issues surface and need to be handled. This does mean that the energy that we balance now never needs to be worked on again because there is no engine to re-stick the energy. Stuck energy once freed stays free! This is a blessing. Every body responds differently to this process.

## What Does a Detox Reaction Feel Like?
### (The Proof of the Healing Happening)

After this process is experienced the cells in your body dump out toxins. This is just a fact of cells and healing. When cells are traumatized they hold onto toxins to fill the hole left there by pain. A detox reaction might be profound tiredness for a day or two. It is as if you can't even get out of bed. This is because your body is using 100% of its energy to heal. You can push past this healing but why would you do that? You waited all your life to reach this healing point. Let the healing happen.

You can get your work, projects, and "stuff" done later/tomorrow. We suggest you get plenty of rest/sleep, take "B" and "C" Complex vitamins, and drink a lot of water to flush the toxins out of your body.

Detox can also be disorientation, lack of depth perception, nausea, dizziness, having the "runs," uncontrollable crying/grief, etc. Sometimes past pain will surface, it will feel the same as it did originally, and it will dissipate and go away in a day or two. Please be careful when you are driving after sessions and realize that your depth perception may be affected. Leave plenty distance around you and other cars on the road. Take surface streets and drive slower than usual if necessary. Please feel free to call this office if the detox reaction gets too great. The greater the release, the greater the detox reaction.

# DEFINITION of HEALING:

Healing is defined as wholeness, balance, connection, ease, things flowing and working properly in your body. Your body has more energy in it than you think. Flowing energy heals, and stuck energy causes issues where it is stuck. It's all about flow and flowing energy. Past memories of trauma can stick flow. Those memories can be freed up. This method frees up that stuck energy in a group. There are processes to free stuck energy in individuals. Once I started doing this work I realized how abused some of us were when we were young. Some people escaped youth unscathed.

There can not be wholeness with random, unaligned or unbalanced energy in the body. Healing is flowing balanced energy. Things work well. Some people have energy going every which way but aligned and flowing.

Energy that moves freely in the body heals as it moves.

Energy that is stuck can cause health issues.

I have met people that have balls of stuck energy in their heart, lungs, brain and/or stomach areas.

Interestingly enough, they also have a lot of health issues in these areas.

I have several friends that died 15 to 30 years younger than I was. Their loss inspired the research and writing of this healing method.

# Instructions for the Facilitator-Presenter

- This is a fun, close, caring, positive, healing community process. It is kept "light" and easy to do. Tell the participants that everything you say and have them do is positive, supportive and, helpful. You will not have them do anything that is not supportive.
- Ask the participants to help you throughout the process coordinate the people in the group so that it goes smoothly.
- Your job is to coordinate, to inform, to keep the process moving along, and to inspire, if possible.
- It is important to read through this section and the process to remind you to stick to the script because it works.
- When you find things that work really well, please email this office with your findings. Your input is very important to us.
- Have your group form a circle holding hands, facing center and standing shoulder to shoulder.
- It is okay to have two, three or more circles inside each other in a large group.
- Have the group feel the energy of the circle and in the group because it is going to change very fast.
- Have the group let their hands go and turn to their right, toward "Your partner's back".
- The person to your right is your partner during this process.
- Let the people know that they can leave the group any time they wish, and tell the others to automatically tighten up the group so all are still

connected during the process. There does need to be enough room for the people to move closer if need be. People will leave the group during the process. Be ready for that.

- If people chose not to participate, that is totally fine.
- Tell the group that the process will go ten minutes and that you will time the event with a timer. Kitchen timers that ring seem to work the best. Timing is precise because of the intensity of the healing energy.
- Do not go past the ten minutes.
- Some of the people in the circle have never had these positive words said to them. It can be emotional.
- Important: Some people have mobility issues, they can sit on chairs in the circle if necessary, it is okay to place one's hands on their partners waist, outside hips or outside thighs if the heart area is too difficult to reach. Always two hands on your partner. The holding wish/prayer goes to the partners' heart wherever they hold.
- Some people prefer to place both hands on top of, or to the sides of their partners shoulders. This is fine as long as the connection remains.
- It is recommended that you only do the process for ten minutes at a time. The group can take a fifteen minute break and then do the process again. Always take breaks after each ten minutes of "circle healing time." You use a kitchen timer or a time keeper to do timing. Timing is precise. Ten minutes at a time max. This is because the healing energy is intense.

The group is a microcosm of the world, and it's energy.

- This is so key for you the facilitator to know; There will be a point where people just start leaving the circle. You might think; "Oh! No!" "Everything is falling apart!" and "What did I do wrong?"

  Relax! And take a deep breath! Your group is a success!

  People are dropping out because the energy got too intense, and they are complete on that part of the process! All participants are free to leave whenever they feel like it. Once a quarter of the group drops out you know it is time to end off. Even if the ten minutes are not up.

- Showing care and love is healing in itself. In a group it has power.

- Even though this process is light and fun to do, it can be intense. People may burst into tears or express other emotions. This is a release and that is good.

  Reassure the group that all is well and continue.

# The Healing Circle Process

You the facilitator say to the group;

- "Say to your partner: I support your healing and my healing enough to work on you for the next ten minutes!"
- "Ask your partner: Is it okay for me to work on you?"
- "Please wait for their response."
- "Please affirm: I will not touch any sensitive parts of your body. This is for our healing."
- "Please wait for their response."
- "Then place both your hands on your partner's back heart area at the left and right scapula."
- "This is important: Keep both hands on your partner during the whole process. This is the heart area. Four to six inches apart is good."

Read one phrase at a time and have them repeat it to their partner.

- "Say to your partner; I am holding your heart in my hands,
- and I am loving you and your heart,
- and I am caring for you and your heart,
- and I am healing you, and your heart, and your life"
- "I want you and your tribe to be well and to be healed."


- "Your heart is so full of love,

16

- "You have so much love to give,"
- "I am holding your heart energy still so that it can heal."
- "I am holding this groups' heart energy still so that they all can heal."
- "The energy in this group is healing energy,"
- "It is as if every person in the circle is working on you, and I, and as well as on each other!"
- "Say to your partner; "I want the same healing done for myself and for my tribe,"

- "Here's the treat!!! Feel the heat or the cool rise/increase your partner, and in the room ( ▲ )! That is the energy of our 'tribe' balancing, it's their energy healing them and all of us! It goes around the circle. The longer you do the process the healing energy becomes stronger."

- "Now we will ask your angels, ancestors, masters, guides, family, and friends (and past pets if you wish) to join the circle now. Past pets were comforters and they are welcome."

(Have the group feel the energy in the circle change when the ancestors, etc. enter.)

- Now, ask your saints, and all the Great Healers of all time to join the circle. Saint Anthony, Saint Theresa, Saint Germain, Saint Francis, Mother Theresa, Mother Mary, Jesus the Healer, Buddha the Healer, Diana, the Princess of Wales, Nelson Mandella, and all the others, (you can name your own healers here).

Have the group feel the energy in the circle change when these healers enter.

Then say this to the group;

- "It is their energy!"
- "This is new information!"
- "The rising heat in this room is the group releasing energy!"

## About five minutes into the process have the group do these affirmations;

You, the leader, say the affirmation and have the group participants repeat them to their partner,
Please allow an appropriate pause between each line;

- You are a wonderful person, (the group repeats it.)
- You are beautiful, or handsome, (lady or man)
- You are decent, kind and honest,
- You are amazing,
- You are awesome,
- You are light,
- You are unconditional love,
- Thank you for being here today and helping,
- You are so worth this healing process,
- You are wisdom,
- You are healing,
- You are an amazing healer,
- You are such a valuable being,
- You have such tremendous gifts for this world,

- You are the healing you want to see in the World,
- Wherever you go people are healed by your presence,
- You are a brilliant miracle worker,
- I am amazed by all the Light coming from your body!
- I am amazed by all the Light coming from your head,
- I am amazed by all the Light coming from your heart,
- I am amazed by your awesome wonderfulness!
- Thank you for being my partner,
- and thank you for allowing me the gift of working and healing with you!
- By the power vested in me by the Universe,
- I forgive you now for all your wrong-doing,
- I forgive you now for all your mistakes and errors,
- I forgive you now for all your crimes known and unknown,
- I forgive you now for all your shortcomings and sins,
- I forgive your ancestors, masters and guides now for all their wrong-doing,
- I forgive you now for all your _____
  (insert what you wish)
- I love you,
- You are a blessed, wonderful being of Light,
- I honor you,
- I respect you,
- I really like you,
- I hold you in high esteem,

- People really like you, and I can understand why,
- Thank you so much for being you,
- Thank you for being here and helping us,
- Thank you for bringing your angels, ancestors, family, saints and healers here today,
- I bless every step and every breath you take,
- I ask all the great healers of all time to use my hands for all of our healing now.
- Come Saint Germain,
- And the Violet Flame and heal this group,
- Come Saint Theresa and heal this group,
- Come Holy Spirit and heal this group,
- Come Jesus, Mary and Joseph and heal this group,
- Come Saint Anthony, and Saint Francis and heal this group,
- Come Archangel Raphael, also known as "the healer" and heal this group,
- You and your ancestors and family are healed,
- You and your angels and masters are healed,
- You and your guides, and past pets are healed,
- You and your community and the world is healed…

Then say to the group; "For one minute we are going to do this; Please keep your hands on your partner and lean close to them and whisper all the things that you wished your parents would have said to you when you were a child… If you can't think of anything to say, just say; 'I love you, thank you for being you, you are so wonderful, please forgive me' and repeat that over and over."

(Continued on next page)

## When the Ten Minutes Are Up Say;

- It is okay to celebrate the release of this stuck energy!
- This stuck energy is better out of you than in you!
- If you wish to continue in the circle of healing take a fifteen minute break and come back.
- If you wish to work in pairs, you are welcome to do so.
- If you wish to just watch, that's fine, too!
- If you wish to just leave, please buy the books that you need and start doing this community healing process in your area.
- Thank you all for being a part of this healing circle.
- Please come back next week for more.

"Thank you all for your participation!"
"This ends this session."

"You can get copies of this book at Amazon, or your local bookstores. We need a lot of people doing this process to shift the energy of the world."

"Thank you for being a part of this healing."

When the group breaks up the people are in a different state than when they started. Be careful of what you ask them to do. You can ask them to sign an email or contact list, volunteer their time to help you, or whatever. Do not take advantage of their vulnerability. Remind them that if they are driving or going up or down stairs that their depth perception will be "Off." And to be careful and to leave a lot of room around themselves and other cars on the road.

This author is creating a team of
facilitators that are willing to use this
community healing process to shift the
energy of this planet.
A "Team Planet Healing" as it were.
You are welcome to join today.

# Prove to Me that Cell Memory is Real!

About 25 years ago a little 10 year old girl needed a heart transplant. When another little girl was murdered, the girl on the transplant list got the heart of the dead girl.

The transplant girl started having these horrible nightmares of being killed. The parents sent their daughter to a psychiatrist. After months of therapy the psychiatrist concluded that this was not bad nightmares, but recall. This was because the "dream" never changed and the details were vivid. A report was sent to the police, and the person who did the murder was arrested and convicted on the heart transplant girl's information. The information in the heart was that accurate.

Sends chills down one's spine, doesn't it?
Other transplant recipients who formerly only listened to rap music, start listening to classical music. Others who had no musical talent or training would, after the transplant, take up playing the piano, flute, violin, or cello! People who had fear of heights would take up extreme rock climbing after a kidney or liver transplant. These stories are searchable on the Internet under "transplant recipient recall."

Cells do hold memory of trauma in them. This process works, and you need not believe any part of this to experience the healing from this work.

We are spiritual beings.

The spirit needs healing, too.

The Four Healing Quadrants are the

Four Keys Necessary for Healing to be

Complete.

This Complete Healing System is a gift,

And it is for your use.

# The Four Healing Quadrants,
4 Keys Necessary for Healing to be Complete.
We are spiritual beings.
The spirit needs healing, too.

| | |
|---|---|
| **Angels & Ancestors,**<br>**Including the Spirit** | **A Workable Healing Method** |
| **Grounding** | **Forgiveness** |

Finally the four keys to complete healing have been discovered. This is a healing breakthrough. Each quadrant represents 25% of the complete composition of healing.

## Do You Only Want to Heal Twenty-Five percent?

Do you only want to heal only Twenty-Five percent (25%)?
How about Fifty percent (50%)? Is that good enough for you?
When all four of these elements are present, real healing can take place. Here's the big value secret; You can implement these four keys today into any and all healing modalities and get better results than you are getting now. Even surgeries, even allopathic, even dentistry, homeopathic, Chinese herbs and acupuncture, chiropractic, Ayurvedic, and energy, etc. healing. The spirit-plus-the-physical does a better job of healing than does all the other methods combined. All healing methods are valid. They all work better when the spirit is included. We energy healers all work on the same energy. It's just how we resolve stuck energy that is different. This is a fast group healing method. That makes it different, unique, valuable and useful. All the training one needs is in this book.

# Considering You, the Spirit in Your Own Healing

All healing goes better/quicker when you and your angels and ancestors are included.

# Angels & Ancestors

We heal together as a tribe or group. When your tribe heals - you heal. Your tribe includes your angels, ancestors, family and friends, masters and guides, and past pets*. They may have not had the opportunity to heal that which might have killed them. Don't look now but your DNA is a protein code linking you to your ancestor's health issues. That DNA code has their and your health information in it, including their pain and health issues. You can believe it or not. Your belief system changes nothing because that's how it works. Future medical research will bear this out.

\* Past pets were and are healing and comforting guides to you and they are included here. Pets need healing, too, because they have similar nervous systems and traumas.

# A Workable Healing Method

I don't know any people that say; "I only want to heal fifty percent, half-way." Every cell in your body responds to spiritual energy, this is because life is connected to spirit. Healing is a spiritual event. When one looks at healing as a physical event, that is like being at the ocean, looking intently at a grain of sand, and not seeing the ocean. Healing must address the spirit. Having a workable healing method is such a blessing. It saves you the trouble of; "not having to re-invent the wheel!" And all you have to do is just learn it and do it. People in the healing arts respect methods that work consistently. This healing system works consistently. Try it and you will see. I tell people; "You need to feel it to believe it." It works that well. This author is very suspect of any healing system that does not consider the spiritual side of healing. You have to love and respect the people in your life enough to want to make a difference in their health. This method may be the only place they can get this health balancing help. And it depends on you and your decisions, care and commitment to this work. Someone else just might not come along and do it. It's up to you. Even the medical arts would benefit from implementing these principles of these healing quadrants in their practices and protocols.

> **For example a surgeon could say; "Before I make this first incision, I am asking this person's angels, guides, masters and ancestors to guide my hand, and to be a part of this healing. It is okay for this tribe to heal together with this person."**
> **Try it and see the results.**

28

# Grounding

Grounding is so important to healing. When we lived in primitive tribes we walked barefooted, in contact with the ground. Now we live and work in buildings that are above ground. Unless we walk on damp grass barefooted, or barefooted on the ground, or swim in a pool or in the ocean, we rarely are grounded. A good one quarter of healing is grounding. One can get a grounding strap as is used in computer work and wears it daily for staying grounded, and especially during healing. Ground is the ultimate balance. A good solid physical ground helps one connect spiritually. Remember that the Buddha sat on the ground and meditated to become enlightened. There is no greater holistic healing than grounding yourself. Even organic nutrition (important) and clean (ecological non polluting – non toxic) living is second to grounding.

# Forgiveness

Forgiveness has gotten a bad rap in the past. People may hate the concept of forgiveness because it is misunderstood.

They can do all of the above healing steps except for forgiveness. This limits their healing. My years of working this method with people has shown the failure or unwillingness to forgive holds people's pain in place. Why would one deliberately clip their healing wings by 25%?

On forgiveness one does what one can, realizing that it may take time to completely forgive. One can face a mirror daily and say; "I forgive myself and others that have wronged me." You may or may not believe it. It doesn't matter. Just do it. Over time it will become easier to forgive. The phrase; "Forgive and forget" might be better expressed, "Forgive, and learn form the past, and be careful in the future."

# Would You Benefit from this Healing Technique?

1. Have you ever fallen more than three feet to the ground? Or have you had other severe falls, like down stairs, out of trees, off roofs, off fences, off cliffs, off horses, off ladders, off bicycles, trips and falls?
2. Have you ever been hit in the head with a ball, rock, or other hard object, even accidentally during sports?
3. Have you ever played football or other sports where head injuries can happen?
4.  Have you ever been hit by a baseball bat or hockey stick to the head or body, even if accidental?
5. Have you already had a stroke, heart attack, cancer, etc. where your life was threatened? *(*Important Note: There is no representation here that this process can fix these issues. The damage is done. This process can balance stuck energy associated with these events.)
6. Have you ever been severely beaten?
7. Have you ever had broken bones or painful surgeries?
8. Have you ever been in an auto or plane accident/crash?
9. Have you ever been confined for long periods of time?
10. Have you experienced any abuse as a child sexually, or otherwise?
11. Have you ever been enslaved, starved, tied up and punished, drugged, shunned or emotionally abused?

12. Have you ever had a bad drug trip? Overdose, etc.?
13. Have you ever been shot or shot at?
14. Have you ever been in a combat zone as a soldier or as
    a civilian?
15. Have you ever had a life altering trauma, emotional or
    physical?
16. Have you ever had nerve issues or disorders?
17. Have you ever been in a coma?
18. Do you suffer from chronic pain?
19. Are you on pain medication?
20. Do you suffer from unexplained pain?
21. Do parts of your body creek or hurt when you get up in the   morning?
22. Have you ever lied to your doctor about having pain?
23. Have you ever been told; "Your pain is all in your head?"
24. Do you suffer from unexplainable chronic life conditions?
25. Do you avoid people at all costs?
26. Are you alone in a crowd?
27. Do you have few or no friends?
28. Are you depressed most of the time?
29. Do you have no interest in life?
30. Do you hate your life, or resent your being victimized?

If you answered "Yes" to any three or more of these questions then you could possibly benefit from doing this healing method, that is after you discuss these issues with a qualified medical professional and you get help. This method balances early cellular memories of pain/trauma. The cells remember pain when you have forgotten. Huge healing issues can resolve with this method. It's worth the price of this book and it's worth the effort to learn and to do this method. You are worth the time. You are worth the effort. And you are worth the healing. This method can not hurt, and it can only help. It's like vitamins, if you don't need them you feel nothing, and if you do need them they are like miracle, life-helping supplements. It's worth a try.

This author is searching for the 100th Monkey (energetically), and he needs Your help by having you start and run healing groups in your community!

# The Story of the 100<sup>th</sup> Monkey

A story about social change.  By Ken Keyes Jr.

The Japanese monkey, Macaca Fuscata, had been observed in the wild for a period of over 30 years.

In 1952, on the island of Koshima, scientists were providing monkeys with sweet potatoes dropped in the sand. The monkey liked the taste of the raw sweet potatoes, but they found the dirt unpleasant.

An 18-month-old female named Imo found she could solve the problem by washing the potatoes in a nearby stream. She taught this trick to her mother. Her playmates also learned this new way and they taught their mothers too.

This cultural innovation was gradually picked up by various monkeys before the eyes of the scientists. Between 1952 and 1958 all the young monkeys learned to wash the sandy sweet potatoes to make them more palatable. Only the adults who imitated their children learned this social improvement. Other adults kept eating the dirty sweet potatoes.

Then something startling took place. In the autumn of 1958, a certain number of Koshima monkeys were washing sweet potatoes -- the exact number is not known. Let us suppose that when the sun rose one morning there were 99 monkeys on Koshima Island who had learned to wash their sweet potatoes. Let's further suppose that later that morning, the hundredth monkey learned to wash potatoes.

# Then It Happened!

By that evening almost everyone in the tribe was washing sweet potatoes before eating them. The added energy of this hundredth monkey somehow created an ideological breakthrough!

But notice: A most surprising thing observed by these scientists was that the habit of washing sweet potatoes then jumped over the sea... Colonies of monkeys on other islands and the mainland troop of monkeys at Takasakiyama began washing their sweet potatoes.

Thus, when a certain critical number achieves an awareness, this new awareness may be communicated from mind to mind.

Although the exact number may vary, this Hundredth Monkey Phenomenon means that when only a limited number of people know of a new way, it may remain the conscious property of these people.

But there is a point at which if only one more person tunes-in to a new awareness, a field is strengthened so that this awareness is picked up by almost everyone!

From the book "The Hundredth Monkey" by Ken Keyes, Jr. The book is not copyrighted and the material may be reproduced in whole or in part.

Read the whole book.

Healing Authors' Notes;  http://www.wowzone.com/monkey.htm

The 100th Monkey Theory has been on the "Wowzone" site since 1996, and we occasionally receive letters claiming that it was a hoax or fake.

We contacted Penny Gillespie, who was married to Ken Keyes and participated in his work and writing. Here is her response:

I'm not sure what you mean by "fake." The Hundredth Monkey is a real book and hundreds of thousands of copies were printed and circulated, often through university courses. People bought them by the case and gave them away.

The story of the hundredth monkey came from a writing by Rupert Sheldrake.

After our book was printed, there was some question about whether the study was authentic. Ken presented the story as a legend, or phenomenon; the concepts of morphogenetic fields and critical mass are very true and the story serves to illustrate them.
I hope that answers your question.

All the best,

Penny Gillespie
President's Club, Platinum Wellness Consultant
www.5Pillars.com/pennygillespie

## This Author's Guarantee to You:

Besides continuing to give you workable healing methods, and my commitment to relentless research for healthy things that work, I guarantee that I will give you technical support on this healing system as long as you need it. Call me before you do a group meeting and tell me you need support on a certain day and between certain times. When you call I will be there for you to answer any questions. There is no need to stay stuck!  (408) 253-6577, Our healing center is in Cupertino, California, U.S.A., near Apple Computer.

## What this Author Needs from You!

Most communities have movers and shakers that are working to make people better. Please find the five most active community leaders in your area and give them a copy of this book. Please ask them to do the process with their groups. Please, also take this process into your communities and where ever you can gather a group of people, churches, community organizations, clubs, family and friends gatherings, reunions, etc.. Please use this process to heal them. As your communities heal, the collective energy of this world will shift. When we reach the critical mass, like the "Hundredth Monkey," then our society's consciousness will shift and real global healing will take place. Maybe we can build a better world for ourselves and for our children.

The intention behind this book is to get copies into the hands of the national representatives at the United Nations in New York. This intention can also be extended to all leaders as well as all governing bodies. This author believes that when these leaders take this healing method to their own countries, and they do the process regularly, we collectively can produce the needed healing shift much faster. People wishing to contribute to this campaign are welcome to contact this office and we can discuss the possibilities. We also need volunteers.

Please also buy ten copies of this book and give them to community and church leaders, as well as healers and people in the wellness professions. This will help in the push to get this information out into the world.

If you are good at proofreading or editing, and you send me a marked up copy of this book, as long as the suggestions are significant, I will mail you five (5) books in return. I can really use your help on this. This offer is good now and for up to one year from March 1, 2014.

# This Author is "Social Media Challenged."

This author is "Social Media Challenged." Please post news of this healing process on Twitter, Facebook, Tumblr, Instagram Pinterest, Linkedin, Pinterest, Google Plus, and even MySpace, Tagged, and all the others, and create buzz and awareness.

If you wish to donate your time to help this organization we can use all the help we can get. This is a volunteer position because we have a limited budget. Donating money, cars, and/or real estate is also appreciated and the funds keep us working.

# Working on a PBS Special!

You are a gold mine of ideas! I need ideas for this PBS special to present this process to the world!
If you have any ideas for this PBS special, please jot them down for me and email them to this office. Please be sure to add your name, email address and phone number. Our **email address** is; <u>healingangelguides@yahoo.com</u>;

Also, we are targeting a budget for this special of $250,000. We need all the donations we can get to create this special. We have a creative team in place ready to produce this special. We just need the funds.

## I Need Ideas for These:

- A title for this PBS Special about community healing
- A book title to accompany this PBS Special
- A title for a book about Angels
- A title for a book about honoring and healing Ancestors

Thank You for your help on this.

# How to Become a Healing Rock Star

We have a healing club that we call our "Healing Rock Stars."

Our Healing Rock Stars are the people that take this work so seriously that they rock the world of others by doing this community healing process with a hundred groups or more.

This work takes dedication, care, and drive. The results are worth it. Our goal is to motivate over one thousand new people a year to become Healing Rock Stars.

**Q:** So what does one needs to do to become a Healing Rock Star?

**A:** One needs to write a report on each group healing after each session and put the date, location, size of the group, the results one got, plus any issues that may have surfaced during the sessions. These reports need to be sent to our office for review. Please email us for our address, and send only copies of your reports to guard against loss in the mail. One sheet of paper per report, please. Make each report as detailed as you can. This gives us valuable feedback.

In the future we are planning events for our Healing Rock Stars.

# Permission to Copy this Book

There is bulk pricing available from this office that often can rival the cost of copying. Please call for bulk pricing.

Permission to copy this book is based on several conditions being met. Our intention is to get this work out into the world and to be widely used. Please call this office for further information, **(408) 253-6577** and tell us of your intention to do that.

Otherwise: All rights reserved.

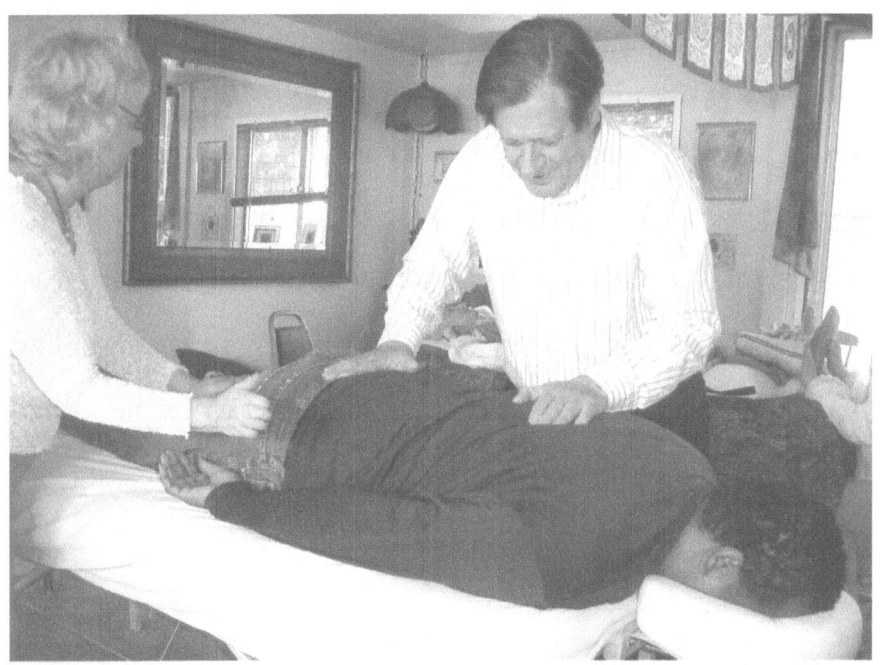

This photo is of our healing center in Willow Glen, part of San Jose, California. In the photo is Paul Barbaro, his wonderful assistant Mona Angel, and a client named Robert.

## Bio of author, Paul Barbaro

Paul Barbaro is an author of four books, speaker, health researcher, and longevity coach. He studied Psychology, languages, education and has a BS degree from UC Riverside, California.

Paul is an "Angel Whisperer." Paul channels your angels to help in your healing. He is an avid medical researcher.

His strength is that he knows what he is looking for and does not quit until he finds it. Paul's persistence keeps him looking only for those things that work consistently well. Paul's healing system was given to him by two Native American (First Nation) Indian shamans. Paul had a thriving healing practice in 2008, and when he added this healing system to his practice, his healing results and client satisfaction went through the roof!

Paul continues his research and healing work in Cupertino, California, near Apple Computer, and people interested in Paul's healing magic can call and make appointments. One does need to come to California, and stay for awhile. Healers that have a practice or spa can learn to do this healing system and boost their results and client satisfaction. There are training classes available in California. Paul presents informative, entertaining, enlightening, and captivating talks, lectures and presentations! Please call to book Mr. Barbaro for your next event.

It is okay for you to donate to us to help keep our healing mission going. Please consider us for your charity giving.

**Our Donation Hotline Toll <u>FREE</u> Phone Number:**

# 1 (800) 500-6540

We can accept donations from all over the United States. We can use cars, SUV's, trucks, real estate, trusts, stock and trading accounts, boats, RV's, timeshares, jewelry, coin and stamp collections, antiques, and anything of value. We are applying for tax exempt status and we appreciate your support and donations. Please use this number for donations only as each call costs us money.

www.ingramcontent.com/pod-product-compliance
Lightning Source LLC
Chambersburg PA
CBHW030535290526
45786CB00004B/1721